ESSENTIAL OILS GUIDE

Essential Oils For Weight Loss, Stress Relief, Aromatherapy, Beauty Care

Easy Recipes For Health & Beauty

MIRANDA ROSS

TABLE OF CONTENTS

The World of Essential Oils

I want to thank you and congratulate you for purchasing the book "Essential Oils Guide: Essential Oils For Weight Loss, Stress Relief, Aromatherapy, Beauty Care. Easy Recipes For Health And Beauty".

The world of essential oils is very fascinating. You are to about to begin your journey with the wonderful Essential Oils. A whole new world of promise awaits you. "Essential Oils" is perhaps nature's most powerful forms in aromatic liquid. Essential oils are extracted from different varieties of flora, fruits, leaves, shoots and barks of trees.

This book will point you towards the direction of holistic healing, so you would have the arsenal to use it as a tool for healing, beauty, weight loss and rejuvenation. You will be introduced to the basics of essential oils – what it is, what it can do, how and how you can use it to your advantage. This book intends to provide essential information to spike your interest and to infuse the benefits of Essential oils in your life.

Thanks again for purchasing this book, I hope you enjoy it!

The trademarks that are used are without any consent, and the publication of the trademark is without permission or backing by the trademark owner. All trademarks and brands within this book are for clarifying purposes only and are the owned by the owners themselves, not affiliated with this document.

DISCLAIMER: The purpose of this book is to provide information only. The information, though believed to be entirely accurate, is NOT a substitution for medical, psychological or professional advice, diagnosis or treatment. The author recommends that you seek the advice of your physician or other qualified health care provider to present them with questions you may have regarding any medical condition. Advice from your trusted, professional medical advisor should always supersede information presented in this book.

Chapter 1: Introduction To Essential Oils

Essential Oils are perhaps one of the most underutilized resources available in nature. For centuries the world over, full-bodied concentrates of many herbs, flowers, plants and fruits were distilled for consumption. The power of these ancient potions is forgotten in modern times. Instead we prefer to consume products with chemicals that mimic the innate aroma of these oils.

Essential Oils are fragrant and sweet smelling. Most people assume that their value lies in its charm and fragrance. But they seem to be mistaken. Modern research indicates that essential oils are powerful and have remarkable medicinal properties. Complex in their molecular arrangement these concentrates are very intense and powerful.

These wonderful liquid concentrates are indispensable to consumables, pharmaceutical and beauty industries. Today about 300 different types of Essential Oils constitute a highly effective system of medicine. Some are popular ingredients in drugs or have become the stimulus for chemical duplication.

Cosmetic manufacturers appreciate their beauty enhancing and cell-rejuvenating properties. The aroma industry is concerned about delightful smells and their emotion augmenting capacities. Each type of oil can have diverse purposes. The single oil can have far reaching benefits. The same oil can be used as anti-inflammatory, treat arthritis and rheumatism and can be prescribed by for discomfort in the digestive system.

Essential oils are not retained in the body unlike chemical drugs. They leave no toxic residue. The air is cleansed by essential oils because they alter the molecular composition and create new smells instead of concealing the unwanted. It is a brilliant alternative to harmful products in our homes and lives. Essential oils offer a convenient, pleasant and practical solution.

These extremely precious liquids are extracted from distinctive varieties of plants and help restore balance and bring harmony is people. With the use of essential oils we not only provide protection from chemicals for ourselves but also the environment.

Essential oils are liquids that are usually extracted in a process called distillation. Distillation is a widely-used technique in which elements of a substance or a liquid mixture are separated from one another by condensation or evaporation. In getting essential oils, liquids are extracted from the stems, leaves, bark, roots and flowers of a plant.

Some would mistakenly think that essentials are the same as perfumes. While essential oils are derived from natural plants, perfume oils are artificial and are comprised of artificial elements. Perfume oils do not have the therapeutic advantages which essential oils can offer.

The History of Essential Oils

Essential oils have had an interesting and colorful history. In recorded history they have been around for ages. Egyptians are credited with the discovery of this ancient medicine. Evidence of this is found on scrolls dating back to 1500 B.C.

There are Biblical references as well. There was a chapter elaborating the practice of worship using these aromatic oils. The wise men were bearing myrrh and frankincense.

Around 500 BC, the Arabs were leading in the trade. The famous he distillation process and administered them extensively. Romans and Greeks were widely believed to have benefitted from the consumption of these oils. Hippocrates, the Father of Medicine, is believed to have used them to stop the spread of plague in Athens. Another prominent Greek physician Dioscorides has authored a book describing methods that are still in use and referenced by modern aroma therapists. Many well-known historical figures like Cleopatra, Napolean and Alexander the Great have said to make use of these glorious aromatics.

During both the World Wars the use of essential oils was far and wide because of its wound-healing and anti-bacterial components. French doctor Jean Valnet and his student Jean Lapraz discovered that certain disease-causing microbes could not survive in the environment of certain essential oils.

In modern France, Dr. Rene-Maurice Gattefosse was working in is laboratory. His experiment exploded and his hands were burned. He dipped them in lavender oil and the gasification of the tissue of his hands ceased. If not it could have easily resulted in gangrene. This incident became the catalyst for Dr. Gattefosse to study and research the curative nature of essential oils.

The use of essential oils gained prominence in the mid-1980s. Since then it has only grown in its popularity in combating modern-day illnesses. The list of people who use natural remedies is only growing. It reinforces that anything with a strong inherent value will always make its presence known.

What Are 'Essential Oils'?

'Essential oils' are critical, fragrant solution that is condensed from a plant's leaves, flowers, roots, seeds, bark and resins. In case of citrus fruits, these oils are extracted from the rind. They need large quantities of plant materials for extracting oils. It generally takes at least fifty pounds of plant material to make one pound of essential oil. The ratio however can also be surprising-to make a single pound of oil it takes 2,300 pounds of Rose flowers.

There are a many methods in which Essential Oils are extracted from their source. They are extracted both in large and small quantities depending on availability and usage. Most Essential Oils are extracted using the distillation process via water, steam or steam water. Another method of extraction is called a cold press. Another process used is called maceration. The process is used to extract oil from very few plants.

They are considered the essence or the lifeblood of a plant and play an important role in biological vegetation. The essential oil of a plant is responsible for several functions; from their odor to attract pollinating insects to repelling pests, bacteria, and viruses that can harm the plant. Scientifically, essential oils have been proven to contain the innate intelligence and resonant energy of the plant. Due to this it endows them with the same healing power and people who use them benefit from its innate brilliance.

Each Essential Oil contains more than a hundred chemical compounds and almost all have anti-bacterial and anti-fungal properties. Each chemical compound found in Essential Oils has specific characteristics and provide a number of benefits to both the mind and body. Their natural properties provide a more holistic approach to treating various ailments.

Most Essential Oils have therapeutic qualities and some of them are also know to possess cosmetic benefits as well. These oils contain the actual essence of the plant, flower, leaf that they are extracted from. Some Essential Oils are derived from the roots such as ginger oil, some oils are extracted from seeds such as almond, and some of them come from leaves such as eucalyptus, while a few others are extracted from flowers or wood.

One of the main reasons why the use of Essential Oils has gained popularity in the recent years is because it eliminates the risk of side effects to a large extent. Although the veracity and safety of 'Essential Oils' is debated, proper and safe extraction will help in ensuring quality.

How Do Essential Oils Work?

Vegetable oils which are used for cooking have a composition of molecules that do not allow them to penetrate at a cellular level. On the contrary Essential oils are non-greasy with tiny molecules that have the ability of penetrating every cell and administer healing at the most fundamental level. Their structural complexity allows them to pass through the skin and cellular membranes and perform multiple functions with just a few drops.

They are derived from a natural plant source and you will notice that there is no "oily" or greasy spot. On application to the skin it is quickly absorbed and gets into action immediately. Modern science has tried to duplicate the healing capabilities and chemical constituents of essential oils, but has had little success. The man-made versions lack the life force and the intelligence that characterizes essential oils. Most synthetic compositions not only have multiple u side effects—but also prove to be deadly.

Incredible results have been reported with the use of these oils by many people. However, everybody's experience may vary based on diet, lifestyle and family history.

Storage & Care for your Essential Oils

Essential oils do not contain fatty acids. Hence they do not get rancid like other vegetable oils. Ensure that it is protected from degenerative effects of light, air and heat. Keeping them stored in dark glass which is tightly sealed will guarantee that their quality is retained for years.

Essential Oil Tips

- You should always read the label and remember all instructions.
- Keep lid tightly closed
- Do not use essential oils directly onto the skin. Always use with a carrier oil.
- Always test on the Skin before using. Dilute a small amount and apply onto the inner arm. If any redness, burning, itching, or irritations happens stop using the oil immediately.

- Keep essential oils away from eyes. If the essential oil gets into the eyes, immediately flush with large quantity of milk and seek medical intervention.
- If an essential oil is ingested, rinse mouth with milk, and then drink a large glass of milk. Seek medical advice immediately.
- If essential oils are splashed onto skin and irritation observed, for dilution apply carrier oil.
- Don't buy essential oils with dropper tops that have glass or rubber. Essential oils are very concentrated and will turn the rubber to gum and ruin the oil.

Chapter 2: Essential Oils And Aromatherapy

Aromatherapy has its origins in Europe and has been practiced as an alternative form of medicine as early as the 1900's. Pioneers of this old science believed that the fragrances from these oils stimulated nerves. They send impulses to that part of the brain which controlled memories and emotions. Based on your need, the usage of these oils has either a stimulating or a calming effect on the body.

Most people have the fallacy that aromatherapy entails all that has lovely smells like diffusers, perfumes or scented candles. However, this is not true. Aromatherapy refers to the use of plant based essential oils diluted in a complementary solution for therapeutic usage. These oils are mixed with vegetable oils, lotion or alcohol. It can be inhaled, massaged or sprayed in the air.

Although they are quite different, most tend to think that aromatherapy and essential oil is the same. The term "aromatherapy" is often mistaken because people believe that all oils smell good. Many essential of them do not have an appealing smell. Aromatherapy is use of essential oils that can be inhaled or smelled. They provide a versatile vehicle for healing properties.

Nobody can escape the impact of smells and aromas in our lives. Have you observed that when you wake up feeling sluggish and on smelling the aroma of fresh coffee you feel invigorated? Or, how calm you feel after a walk where the scents of cedar or pine fill the air? Your homemade aromatherapy recipes with essential oils can recreate those feelings and elevate your mood. The sense of smell made easy through the olfactory nerves encourages the oils into the body and even if the scent is faint, healing is taking place.

Aromatherapy especially in the use of pure essential oils is extremely useful in enhancing emotional wellbeing. They can help promote positive emotional states and can help in dealing with issues such as fear, grief, anger, or frustration. They instill a sense of tranquility and add to your well being. Aromatherapy can aid a extensive range of ailments; pains, injuries and aches, pains while alleviating discomforts of many health issues. Acting on the central nervous system, it helps anxiety & depression and stress. It soothes, relaxes, uplifts and, stimulates by restoring physical and emotional well-being.

The appropriate oils can have potent results, both on the spirit and the body. Perfumes, fragrance oils, and other artificially made substitutes for pure essential oils do not have the same powerful results. Aromatherapy is not said to cure any diseases on its own but assists the body in finding natural cures by itself.

Methods of Application

The method employed can in many ways affect the kind of results you receive. You must remember that no essential oil should be applied undiluted to the skin. Normal dilution is about 2.5%, or 15 drops of the essential oil to about 1 Oz of the carrier oil.

Aromatherapy Massage: The most common or popular way the oils are typically administered is through a massage. You can choose your essential oil with suitable vegetable oil. Enjoy the benefits of aromatherapy with this often used technique.

Inhalation: It through inhalation that the aromatic compositions of these natural oils affect our central nervous system. Add 5-7 drops to steaming hot water. Cover your head with a towel to capture the steam. Inhale till you stop smelling the oil or the water cools down.

Baths and Showers: Add about 5-10 drops in a tub of hot water and swish to disperse in the water. Alternatively if you like bath salts use a blend of epsom salts, baking soda and sea salt with the oils.

Post a shower; apply 5 to 7 drops to a damp wash cloth and briskly rub all over the body.

You can refer to the list below to create or enhance your well-being with essential oils:

For Relaxation & Peace: Lavender, Sandalwood, Ylang Ylang, Rose, Lemon, Patchouli, Frankincense, Geranium, Cedar wood, Jasmine, Tangerine, Neroli, and Marjoram.

For Stimulation & Invigoration: Basil, Black Pepper, Wintergreen, Sandalwood Bergamot, Rosemary, Verbena,

Spearmint, Sage, Pine, Ginger, Grapefruit, Frankincense and Patchouli,.

For Mental Clarity: Frankincense, Peppermint, Rosemary, Grapefruit, Lemon, Lemongrass, Roman Chamomile, Cinnamon, Orange, Bergamot, Black Pepper, Basil, Eucalyptus, Vetiver, and Ylang Ylang.

For Focus & Concentration: Nutmeg, Lemongrass, Grapefruit, Fennel, Thyme, Bergamot, Basil, Cypress, Cinnamon and Peppermint

For Romance: Rose, Vanilla, Jasmine, Orange, Ylang Ylang, Cassia, Cinnamon, Sandalwood, Vanilla, and Patchouli.

For Joy & Positivity: Clove, Ginger, Orange, Rose, Jasmine, Cinnamon, Sandalwood, Frankincense, Lemon, Bergamot, Fennel, Pine, Myrrh Patchouli and Geranium.

Chapter 3: Essential Oils For Skin Care And Hair Care

Every year, almost 50 billion dollars is spent by Americans on cosmetic products. The beauty and skin care industry is a huge business. This includes everything from soaps and gels anti-aging products, to acne treatments, deodorants and moisturizers. Tons of new rituals are created and introduced into the market, with promises of improved appearance or energizing your face and body. Unfortunately many of them do not always live up to expectations simply because man-made ingredients cannot possess similar healing properties that nature provides with essential oils. In reality the constituents of commercial cosmetic products have repercussions on your health.

The skin is our body's largest organ and acts as a barrier to keep environmental toxins from entering our body. It protects us in winter from the effects of cold, and guards us in summer from the assault of the UV rays of the sun. However, it is actually like a sponge that soaks up everything it associates with. Similarly, when you use cosmetics that are less than healthy or even toxic—all ingredients are absorbed directly into your skin. There has to be a better way to make you look and feel better jeopardizing your health every day.

According to some health experts, our skin and hair is under attack and stress every day. Are you aware that the U.S. Food and Drug Administration (FDA) has a list that contains some 10,000 cosmetic and skin care ingredients that sits in your bathroom which are unsafe. For example, many hair and skin care products contain parabens. A fairly common additive, it penetrates the skin and once in your body, it stays there and slowly damages your system. The FDA estimates that this class of chemical is the most widely used preservatives in skin and hair care products.

Why Make Your Own Beauty Products

There are primarily two reasons for creating your own skin care products with essential oils to pamper your skin. First, the knowledge that you are using all-natural ingredients, free of toxins and chemicals with tremendous benefits. The second, all chemicals are duplicated synthetically and are less effective than natural versions. By doing so you will notice a fantastic difference from the retail products you've been using. Essential oil-based treatments are way more effective than those churned out by cosmetic companies.

Benefits Of Using Essential Oils For Skin Care

- Hastens collagen production
- Improves moisture content in the skin
- Boost the ability of the skin to protect against environmental toxins
- Reduces the effect of free radicals that harm your skin

- Encourages and stimulates skin cell repair & renewal

The easiest and most effective skin and hair care therapies are easy to create. Once you become experienced in creating these easy rituals you can experiment with different essential oils to that suit your personal skin type. This way, your skin can receive the optimum benefits.

Methods For Using Essential Oils For Skin Care

1. Massage oils
2. Body oils
3. Body sprays & facial mists
4. Facial or steam inhalation
5. .facial toners or astringents
6. Facial oils
7. Lotions or creams
8. Bath
9. Bath salts
10. Bubble bath
11. Body scrubs
12. Shower
13. Compress
14. Bath soaps & powders
15. Lip balms

Five Must Have Essential Oils For Glowing Skin

1. **Carrot seed oil**: It is huge benefit for dry, mature, sun-damaged and wrinkled skin. In winter months when skin appears dull carrot seed oil will help infuse moisture. It is good for both oily and dry complexions.

2. **Lavender oil**: It is used for both sensitive and aging skin. It is anti-fungal, antibacterial and anti-inflammatory. Most beneficial for acne, cuts and burns.

3. **Lemongrass oil**: Increases the glow of the skin and detoxifies and helps in regeneration. It is used as a fungicidal astringent and to minimize pores.

4. **Tea tree oil**: It is best for sensitive and oily skin. It helps repair the skin naturally by cleansing and soothing it.

5. **Monoi oil**: The oil is extracted from the Tahitian Monoi plant blooms and helps your skin glow. It has long-lasting moisturizing properties and purifies your skin. It protects the skin from sun and other weather elements.

Essential oils are a great, natural way to get a gorgeous shimmer; use them and enjoy glowing skin. Essential Oils can greatly help promote healthy and lustrous hair. It can reduce dryness and hair loss. Some of them include:

Chamomile:

- Can be used for fine to normal hair
- Gives sheen and Conditions the hair
- Soothes the scalp inflamed from harsh weather conditions
- Aids psoriasis and scaly scalp

Cedarwood:

- Restores oily and dry scalp to normalcy
- Stimulates hair follicles in the scalp for hair growth
- Effective for dandruff & hair loss
- Used as both astringent and antiseptic

Lavender:

- Used for all types of hair
- Treatment for itchy scalp and dandruff
- Controls hair breakage and aids hair growth
- Helps balance the natural oils of the scalp
- Soothes scalp and has a calming effect on the hair

Peppermint:

- Good for Dry hair
- Acts as a stimulant for blood flow to the hair
- Promotes growth of hair by increased circulation

Tea Tree:

- Great moisturizer for the hair

- Keeps the scalp bacteria free
- Unblocks the sebaceous glands and clears dead skin cells

To use essential oils for hair care ensure that it is not applied directly to your hair or scalp. You can mix it with any carrier oil of your choice or it can be diluted with vinegar or floral water.

Essential Oil Hair Care Recipes

Hair conditioner oil

1 large spoon of jojoba/olive or any other carrier oil

3 drops of rose essential oils (or any hair care essential oil)

Directions: Blend the vegetable oil and the essential oil of your choice. Apply this onto hair wet with warm water. Let it rest for 30 minutes or more. Then, wash normally.

Natural lighten hair

1 large spoon of coconut oil (or any other oil)

3 drops of lemon oil

Directions: Blend all ingredients together. Apply this onto dry or wet hair for 1-2 hours or more. Then, wash normally.

Repeat the procedure at least 2 times a week.

Variation: You can add 3 drops of lemon oil to amount of shampoo that you normally use.

Dandruff mix

Add 2 drops each of lavender oil, cedarwood oil, rosemary oil and tea tree oil to 40ml of carrier oil

Directions: Blend all ingredients together. Apply on the scalp for 30 minutes to 1 hour. Then, wash your hair twice.

Dandruff mix 2

1 egg yolk

1 tablespoon of mask or conditioner

3 drops of rosemary oil or lavender oil

Directions: Blend well ingredients together. Apply on the scalp for 30 minutes to 1 hour. Then, wash your hair as usual.

Scented hair: Apply 2 drops of any 'essential oil' to the comb or hairbrush bristles. As the oil acts on your hair the aroma is absorbed.

Essential Oil Body Care Recipes

Coffee Body Scrub

1 large spoon of ground coffee

2 tablespoon of olive oil (or any other oil you prefer)

4-5 drops of orange oil or grapefruit oil

Directions: Blend well ingredients. Apply on your body by doing the massage.

Body moisturizer

Apply 2 drops of any 'essential oil' to amount of your body balm that you normally use

Shower Gel

2 drops of rose oil

2 drops of orange oil

1 teaspoon of shower gel

1 teaspoon of aloe vera juice (optional)

Directions

Blend all ingredients together. Then, use it during washing or bathing.

Chapter 4: Essential Oils For Weight Loss

Essential oils are very supportive in enabling you to lose weight. The ancient wisdom of essential oil therapy for weight loss has no side effects and is not harmful. The oils work on that part of the brain which deals with the feeling of satiety. It also assists with the breakdown and release of unwanted fat & toxins from the body.

Weight loss is a complex issue and many of us struggle with it constantly. Almost all of us want to shed some pounds and get into better shape. Unfortunately we are often confused about the approach to weight loss. Yes, diet control can work but starving yourself in the long run only leads to frustration and failure.

Your desire for weight loss has sent you to try expensive diet plans, rigorous exercises and consume weight loss pills and you are still not happy with the results. You are wondering what else you can do to control the growing waist line or flabby arms. If you have tried everything but still struggling then you need to evaluate your approach towards weight loss.

Feelings of hunger and fullness play a large role in how and when you eat. Both are important factors in regulating your weight. Different triggers impact hunger and fullness. Aromas have a compelling effect on hunger. For example, you find the aroma of baked cookies or the whiff of a chocolate irresistible. Just when you are about to eat you smell gasoline or something you do not like and your appetite is lost. This means that the sense of smell has an impact on your appetite. Certain aromas enhance craving while others reduce it.

Mother Nature has given aromas to most edibles and this could be to create connect with our desire to eat. Essential Oils are nature's gift that can help you to eat healthy and tame your appetite. They can penetrate into the tissues of the body either as vapors or through the skin. Their influence on the nervous system is said have many psychological and physiological mechanisms. Apart from controlling cravings and reducing appetite, they promote weight loss by reducing stress.

Benefits Of Using Essential Oils For Weight Loss

- Helps to control Blood Sugar, cravings and Hunger
- Acts as a natural detox solution
- Decongestion of the Lymphatic system
- Enhances Digestion
- Reduces fluid retention in the body

Use Of Essentials Oils For Weight Loss

They can be used in three ways:

1. **Inhalation**: We stop eating when our brain signals satiety. The right aromas suppresses appetite, curbs cravings and avoids the consumption of extra calories

2. **Topical Application**: You can apply them topically through cellulite wraps, baths and massages. They tighten the skin at thighs, arms and stomach and reduce cellulite

3. **Ingestion**: You can consume them by adding to water or take it as a capsule.

It is recommended that you choose three or more oils for use during the whole day using any of the above methods. It is advisable to carry them on you and use them frequently for effectiveness. When you are tempted to eat or feeling hungry; before you begin eating, open the bottle. Take three whiffs in every nostril breathing in deeply while keeping the other closed.

Close the bottle immediately to avoid diffusing the smell. It is advisable to rotate the essential oils to avoid getting used to a specific one and to maintain its effectiveness. You can inhale several times daily for best results.

Effective Essential Oils For Weight Loss

'Grapefruit': It is known to lessen cravings and decrease insulin. Blood sugar metabolism is regulated by Insulin. A carbohydrate rich diet with the intake of vegetable fats creates insulin resistance with subsequent weight gain. It also curbs cellulite and overeating.

'Lemon': Great for detoxification of the body. The body's filtration system, the liver is stimulated. The polyphenols found in lemon are known to aid weight loss. Leptin & Glucose improved tremendously by lemon polyphenols and hence prevent morbid obesity.

'**Cinnamon**': Cinnamon improves blood sugar levels. High levels lead to portliness and can cause diabetes, Alzheimer's, depression, acne and many other issues. Cinnamon gently detoxifies which boosts immunity.

'**Ginger**': Ginger is good for digestion, controls inflammation and is great for digestion. Inflammation is causes obesity and chronic inflammation is detrimental to your weight loss.

'**Peppermint**': Peppermint is advocated for those who suffer from IBS. It alleviates constipation, bloating and diarrhea. Peppermint diminishes cravings and limits excess eating. For severe weight problems, it suppresses appetite. People prone to overeating know that they are full and it's time they stop eating.

Chapter 5: Essential Oils For Stress Relief

The grind of living in the city and the constant hustle bustle takes a toll on us. From staying up late, to putting in long hours at the office, to getting stuck in traffic during peak hours or attending late night parties, stress is inevitable.

Take a step back and see how being so busy will damage your health – we eat meals on the go and snack on foods that lack essential nutrients. We constantly inhale fumes dirt and grime and are exposed to pollutants. This goes on day in and day out. Because of this lifestyle our bodies susceptible to diseases and we become easily become ill. Our bodies and minds are actually complaining and want to break away from this vicious cycle.

It is no wonder that more and more people are discovering and experimenting with holistic natural remedies. Our bodies have natural healing tendencies and we should maximize its advantage. Scented essential oils enhance healing of body-mind-spirit. Using them is a pure and unadulterated remedy for bad mood, nagging aches and stress alleviation.

Essential oils are very potent in their concentrated form and hence offer relief and reduce stress. When two different essential oils are mixed with carrier oil, the result is far more beneficial in soothing pains and calming the mind.

The benefits of using essential oils has been widely accepted and researched. The European Journal of Preventive Cardiology in a recent study published that using 'essential oils' is beneficial for stress relief. Taiwanese scientists further add that the benefits also broaden to include blood pressure and the heart rate

Benefits Of Essential Oils For Stress Relief

- Has tremendous Healing Qualities
- Builds Immunity
- Mitigates Pain, Cramps and Headaches
- Revitalizes And Invigorates
- Improves Circulation
- Keeps Flu and Colds at bay
- Alleviates Chronic Fatigue

The therapeutic use of essential oils is now a widely acknowledged and extremely effective way to combat stress. Research indicates that the inhalation of essential oils has immediate stress-relieving effects. It enhances the mood, reduces anxiety and aids in strengthening focus and concentration.

Essential Oils can be introduced in your life in several ways. Diffusers aid the release of molecules in the air by heating the oil. Inhalation of different 'essential oils' can lift spirits, encourage creativity, build focus and cleanse your environment of toxins.

'Essential Oils' For Stress Relief

There many easily attainable essential oils that can be used to minimize the symptoms of stress. Listed below are a few essential oils with their stress-reducing features.

Basil: It is derived from the leaves of the herb and has a fresh sweet but spicy aroma. Considered very useful in cases of mental fatigue, burnout or negativity, it improves clarity, concentration and enthusiasm.

Cinnamon This essential oil is taken from the bark with a sweet, warm and spicy aroma. This oil invigorating, abets positivity and is a great weapon in fighting stress and exhaustion.

Eucalyptus: Eucalyptus oil is colorless and its aroma instantly can be used for cooling and head-clearing. Eucalyptus can be used to counter restlessness, confusion and sluggishness. It boosts confidence, restores balance, and enhances vitality. You can use it to sharpen creativity, and understanding and aids regeneration.

Cedarwood: This essential oils increases stability clarifies purpose and builds focus and concentration. This is useful for anxiety, mental strain and worry.

Orange: This essential oil is extracted from the peel of the fruit. Pale yellow in color and has refreshing smell. It is known to be a mental stimulant and fights burn-out, apathy and anxiety.

Lavender: Known to be very versatile oil it has been used for healing since time immemorial. This is colorless/pale yellow oil with a sweet floral scent. Very useful in stressful situations as it reduces anxiety, depression and fatigue, it restores, balance and promotes relaxation & rejuvenation

Rosemary: This is a colourless/pale yellow oil extracted from flowering tops and has a subtle woody scent. It enhances energy, creativity and clarity. Found to be very useful in cases of strain, lethargy, fatigue and overwork.

Grapefruit: Grapefruit appears a pale yellow in color with a fresh citrus smell. It is known as a mental stimulator and can be used to balance mental exhaustion. This oil greatly reduces frustration, improves clarity, instills positivity and is inspirational.

Lemongrass: Lemongrass with a distinct lemony aroma is yellow in color. This oil helps reduce panic and stress and builds concentration and focus.

Pine: This essential oil has a strong refreshing aroma. Pine essential oil is good when under duress. When faced with a lack of confidence it is assuring and provides balance.

Recipes For Stress Relief

Calming Massage Oil

- Petitgrain - 6 drops
- Neroli - 4 drops
- Orange - 5 drops

Put all the ingredients in to about 15 ml carrier oil as per your choice. Now combine them together and shake well. The combination is now ready to massage into musters and back.

Calming and Stress Relief Diffuser Combine

- Lavender - 18 drops
- Roman Chamomile - 12 drops
- Rosewood- 15 drops
- Clary Sage - 10 drops
- Geranium - 12 drops
- Marjoram - 8 drops
- Ylang Ylang - 10 drops

Combine all ingredients in a small glass bowl and mix well. Add in a diffuser of your choice. Now Sit back and enjoy the soothing effect.

Calming Sleep Oil Combine

- 4 drops - Pine
- 4 drops – Melissa
- 4 drops - Marjoram

- 1 drops - Cinnamon

Add all ingredients into about 15 Ml of any carrier oil and mix well. The formula is now ready to be massaged for a great night of refreshing sleep.

Mix all ingredients and use to massage.

Conclusion

The use of essential oils is recorded extensively in many traditional systems of medicine. Over the last few decades, there is a renewed interest in the use of essential oils for holistic well-being. The Essential oils have substantial benefits and increasingly explored for stress relief, weight management and cosmetic value.

Essential Oils are extracted through a distillation process of the many parts of the plant including the bark, leaves, peels, flowers and resin. Their use ranges from medicinal, aromatherapy, stress relief, personal beauty care to house hold cleansers. They are concentrates and have a strong fragrance. When it is oil concentrate the most compelling and healing composites of the plant is condensed in a single potion. By doing this you harness the healing potential of the plant. It becomes a powerhouse of myriad benefits for those who use it.

Go right ahead and experience this glorious gift of Nature!!

Should you find this book extremely of help, sharing it with your friends and loved ones will be greatly valued.

Thank you and good luck!

Check Out My Other Books

Bellow you will find my other books that are popular on Kindle. Simply click on the links below to check them out.

Health & beauty:

Natural Hair Care Guide: How To Stop Hair Loss And Accelerate Hair Growth In A Natural Way, Get Strong, Healthy And Shiny Hair Without Chemicals

Essential Oils For Pets: Essential Oils For Dogs: 40 Safe & Effective Therapies And Remedies To Keep Your Dog Healthy From Puppy To Adult

Anti-Aging Skin Care Secrets: Younger Skin Without Scalpel And Botox. Discover How To Rejuvenate Your Skin Quickly And Maintain A Youthful Appearance

Growing orchids:

Orchids: Growing Orchids Made Easy And Pleasant. The Most Common Errors In The Cultivation Of Orchids. Let Your Orchids Grow For Many Years

Phalaenopsis Orchids Care: 30 Most Important Things To Remember When Growing Phalaenopsis Orchids, How To Give The Best Life To Your Plants

Speed reading guide for beginners:

Speed Reading Guide For Beginners: Get Your Fast Reading Skill The Easy Way. Simple Techniques To Increase Your Reading Speed In Less 24 Hours

You can simply search for the titles on the Amazon website to find them. Best regards!

www.ingramcontent.com/pod-product-compliance
Lightning Source LLC
Chambersburg PA
CBHW062029280526
45787CB00005B/2255